I0440856

Acid Reflux Solutions And Natural Remedies

A Comprehensive Guide on Acid Reflux Diet And Cures With Simple Recipes

By: Brenda Suarez

ISBN-13: 978-1481964609

TABLE OF CONTENTS

Brenda Suarez

Publishers Notes

ISBN-13: 978-1481964609

First Published In United States 2011 And Licensed For Republication By Blue Shift Publishing LLC on December 20, 2012.

Blue Shift Publishing LLC

7950 NW 53rd Street

Miami,

FL 33166

Paperback Edition 2012

BLUE SHIFT PUBLISHING PRESS is a trademark of Blue Shift Publishing LLC.

For information about special discounts for bulk purchases, please contact Blue Shift Publishing Sales Department at 646-312-7900 or publishing@blueshiftpublishing.com

Manufactured in the United States of America

Disclaimer

This publication is intended to provide helpful and informative material. It is not intended to diagnose, treat, cure, or prevent any health problem or condition, nor is intended to replace the advice of a physician. No action should be taken solely on the contents of this book. Always consult your physician or qualified health-care professional on any matters regarding your health and before adopting any suggestions in this book or drawing inferences from it.

The author and publisher specifically disclaim all responsibility for any liability, loss or risk, personal or otherwise, which is incurred as a consequence, directly or indirectly, from the use or application of any contents of this book.

Any and all product names referenced within this book are the trademarks of their respective owners. None of these owners have sponsored, authorized, endorsed, or approved this book.

Always read all information provided by the manufacturers' product labels before using their products. The author and publisher are not responsible for claims made by manufacturers.

DEDICATION

I would like to dedicate this book to my doctor, who worked diligently with me to aid me in coping with, and eventually overcoming my acid reflux. To you I am eternally grateful!

CHAPTER 1- INTRODUCTION

Acid reflux—the words are all too familiar in today's culture. What is it about this health condition that causes such recognition amongst so many people? Perhaps it's the fact that so many of us are flooded with commercials on this condition, just about every day. Perhaps it's the fact that so many people try to self diagnose this condition every time they have a bit of heartburn.

Maybe it's because so many people are actually suffering from this condition that it's almost become common place. Though the instinct of many is to dismiss acid reflux as a seemingly simple condition, it can be a truly difficult one to live with. If you don't get the proper diagnosis and work through an appropriate treatment plan with a medical professional, then acid reflux may literally take over your life.

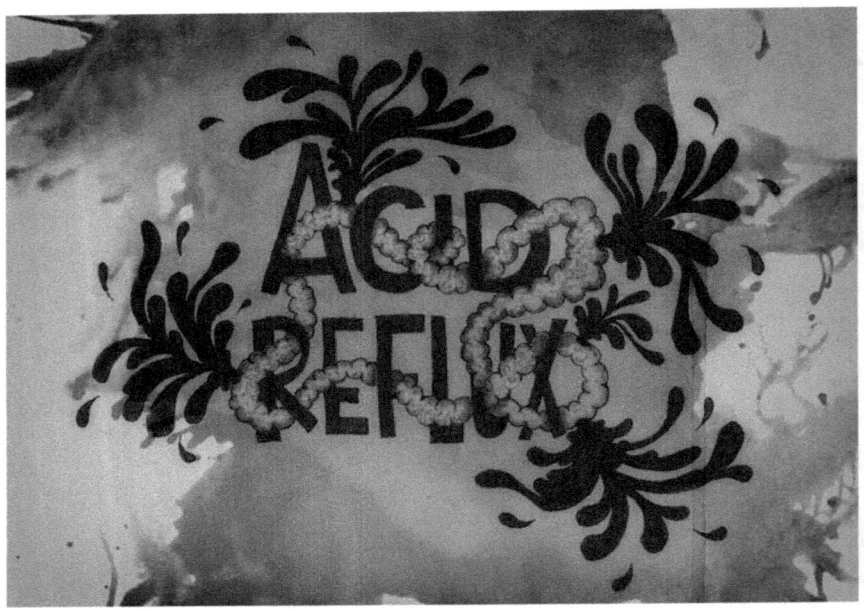

So why is it that acid reflux has become such a common, widespread, and rather accepted health condition? What is it about this particular gastrointestinal disorder that has caused so many to just skip past it? It's hard to say in each individual case, but for the majority it probably has to do with the fact that there are so many different medications out on the market.

So many different drug companies have jumped in on the act to distribute and market their own version of acid reflux medication. You're seeing so many different commercials because there are that many medications that all promise to help you cope with the common symptoms. While this can be a relief to those who suffer from acid reflux and to doctors who prescribe them, it can all be a bit confusing as well.

Understanding what acid reflux is and how to live with it can come in handy. This can be a rather frustrating and debilitating gastrointestinal disorder, and getting into the details of it can help you to coping with it throughout your life.

A COMMON AILMENT POPPING UP EVERYWHERE

What's even scarier is that you hear about acid reflux in some way, shape, or form in just about every segment of the population. Everybody from the very young to the very old seems to be plagued with some level of acid reflux.

Years ago people would have never realized that this seemingly common health condition could cause such unrest amongst so many different segments. It's not uncommon for babies to develop acid reflux or GERD, which is Gastroesophageal Reflux Disease, in reaction to formula or even breast milk. This is certainly something to be taken seriously as babies as young as a few months or even weeks may be put on some form of medication to help them to digest their food.

Though some level of acid reflux has most certainly been around for years, the occurrence has become almost alarming. It seems that people at every age seem to be developing some level of acid reflux and it's inhibiting the simplest functions in their life. No longer can those afflicted with this condition simply eat a meal without suffering. So what is it, where does it come from, and why is it so common these days?

These are all subjects that we will delve into. Understanding how the condition develops and more importantly how it shows up through common symptoms is an important part of the process. Though it's always a good idea to get involved and gain comprehension in any sort of health condition, it is especially true when it comes to acid reflux. Not only can it help with your treatment, but it can help you to cope with it and live with it comfortably.

NOT YOUR RUN OF THE MILL HEALTH CONDITION

Though there are many health conditions that people tend to ignore in their life, acid reflux should not be one of them. If left untreated, this can develop into something more serious which can cause long term damage.

The symptoms may start off simply and slowly but may very well turn into something that becomes almost unbearable to cope with. As we outline what the symptoms are and how they can affect your life, it's important to get ahead of them and do your part to seek out medical attention.

Brenda Suarez

A case of heartburn here and there isn't really the problem, that can happen to anyone. It's when the heartburn begins to occur more frequently and becomes more intense. It's when that heartburn begins to mix with other symptoms and causes the simple act of eating and digesting a meal to seem impossible.

It's when the symptoms of this seemingly simple disease turn into something so complex and overwhelming that it can cause you to think twice before drinking a simple glass of water.

Though everybody is different in terms of their case of acid reflux one thing remains the same—proper diagnosis and treatment is imperative. If you feel that your symptoms are intensifying or multiplying, then get to a doctor. There are a number of different things it could be, but know that acid reflux is something that you can and will live with. If you catch it early on, you can find that certain medications or even lifestyle changes may do the trick.

It's really dependent on what you are willing to do and what changes you are willing to make if this disorder will take over your life. The best thing you can do if you suspect acid reflux or even if you have a family history of it is to get into the doctor to have them take a look.

This does not have to take over your life, and there are some rather simple tools and methods that you can encompass to make it a bit more bearable. Don't give into the frustration and allow this health condition to rule your life.

HELP IS ON THE WAY

We are going to help you every step of the way. We will outline for you the common symptoms of acid reflux. We will tell you what to look for and what it can develop into if left untreated to highlight the sign ficance of this disorder. We will help you to see how medication can help, or perhaps how an alternate treatment may provide aid.

Whi e it's true that acid reflux has become prominent and common amcngst people at all ages and walks of life, it doesn't have to rule you. Part of living with acid reflux is to get educated and to understand what it is and how you can stay ahead of it. Being an educated patient is what will help you not only to get better, but to find a reasonable way to live with it.

Our intention is to educate you and to show you just how you can best cope and live with this often frustrating health condition. Before you let acid reflux rule your life, we will give you the tools to prevent that from happening. Let's get started and figure out what acid reflux is all about.

CHAPTER 2- UNDERSTAND WHAT ACID REFLUX IS

So what really is acid reflux anyway? If you think that the name says it all you are only half right. Yes there is acid involved, but do you know where it come from? Getting a bit scientific and getting into the actual details of this seemingly simple gastrointestinal disorder can be a smart move as a patient who suffers from it.

If you think you know it all or you feel that you can control the symptoms and the condition on your own, then perhaps a proper education is in order. This is not the type of health condition that just pops up as a result of the foods you're eating or the lifestyle you're living.

Though those can be factors in your proper treatment, this is actually a result of an inefficiency in your body. That's why proper diagnosis is so very important and why you must get to the heart of what's really going on.

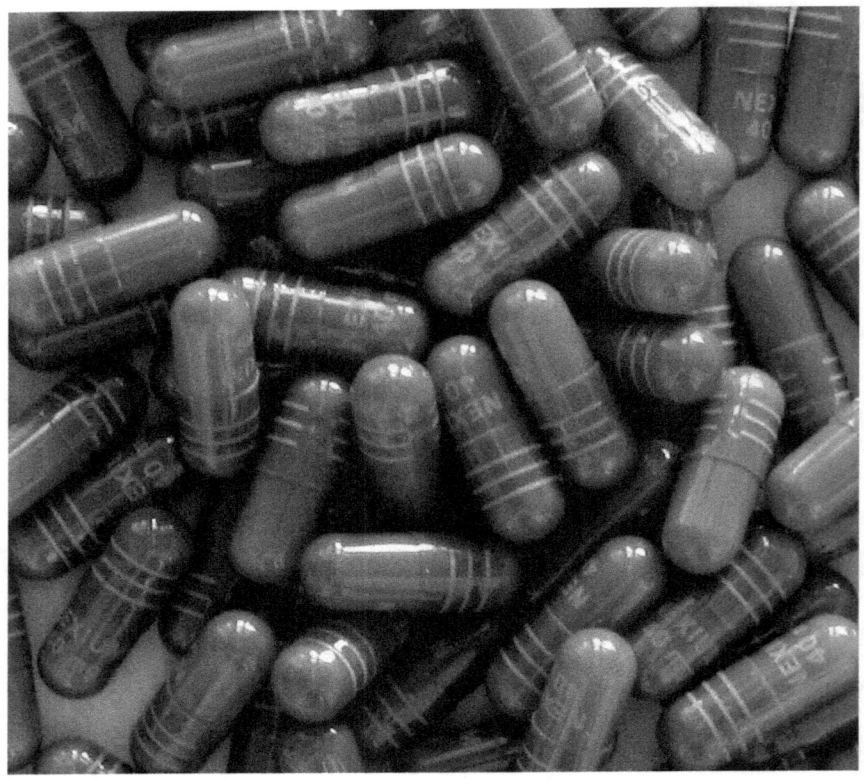

Let's get into the science of it all. Here is what acid reflux derives from:

At the most fundamental level, acids from the stomach flow back into the esophagus. This is what causes the heartburn and that "acidy" feeling in your chest or throat.

The esophagus is the tube between the stomach and the pharynx and it's important to understand its location and importance. This tube is what the chewed food travels through and what is meant to transport it for further digestion. In acid reflux, this is where the problems begin.

The esophageal sphincter is the valve that opens and closes to keep stomach acids from backing up into the esophagus or throat. Normally this valve works properly to keep the stomach acids in the stomach where they aid in the digestion process.

When the esophageal sphincter gets weakened or simply doesn't work properly, this is where the acids can tend to back up. The gastric juices or stomach acid then backs up into the esophagus and then the throat. This is where the pain or burning that many are familiar with comes from, as the acids can produce such results.

In some instances, the esophageal may become weakened and thus contribute to acid reflux later on in life. In other instances, this sphincter may have never developed properly in the first place. This is where you see acid reflux or a related problem occur in babies, where it may be weakened or simply underdeveloped.

UNDERSTANDING HOW IT ALL WORKS

So now you see the science of it all. You understand what exactly is going on in there and why that burning or acidy feeling may come about. It's important to know that people may suffer from some form of acid reflux here and there. Indigestion and heartburn are quite common here and there.

This may be due to certain foods that an individual may eat, or may even come about due to stress. *Some level of acid reflux or heartburn is common and usually if it's an isolated incidence it's nothing to worry about. Here's an easy way to decipher between heartburn and acid reflux—heartburn is the actually sensation or feeling that you suffer from, while acid reflux is the action that causes it.* Acid reflux is the underlying condition that comes about when the acid backs up, and the heartburn is the actual pain that an individual suffers from.

Though it's always a good idea to keep an eye on any sort of heartburn suffered and ensure that it's nothing more serious or associated with a pattern, sometimes heartburn is just heartburn and nothing more. If however you feel like your symptoms are multiplying or intensifying, then you really need to get into a doctor for a proper diagnosis.

While everybody is different, there are some symptoms of acid reflux that can be quite common and even easily recognizable. If you stay ahead of this and educate yourself on the common symptoms it can truly help with diagnosis and ultimately treatment. So here are some of the more common symptoms of acid reflux:

Heartburn: Though we've all suffered from some level of heartburn at one time or another, this is a heartburn that doesn't seem to want to go away. *Remember in this instance, the heartburn may occur more frequently or be far more intense than in an isolated case. This is usually the first symptom and the one to keep an eye on to check for frequency and intensity.*

Pain: Though it may occur anywhere from the stomach and upward with acid reflux, it is most commonly in the throat. The pain may come and go, may be constant, may get worse at times, or may be almost unbearable for those with more severe cases.

Burning: As the acid reflux backs up into the esophagus, this results in a very common burning. In all reality, this stomach acid really does tend to burn. It may come up as a sort of a burping feeling that tends to burn, or it may be a constant and often aggravated burning sensation that doesn't seem to go away at all.

Chest Pain: *This is not usually the type of chest pain that one would confuse with a heart problem, but rather a chest pain that is more annoying and dull in nature. This is often associated with the all too common burning that many complain of with acid reflux.*

Regurgitation: You may start off with an awful taste in your mouth, and this may then turn into a sort of "wet burp". In more severe cases of acid reflux, the regurgitation may even result in vomiting where the food is unable to be digested.

Sore Throat: What may start off with a sore throat that many may mistake for a cold or flu turns into something that is definitely associated with a pain and burning that is unmistaken for a symptom of acid reflux.

Nausea, Bloating, Stomach Discomfort, and Even Vomiting: These are lumped together because if a case of acid reflux gets really intense, then you may see some of these more extreme symptoms come about. *The confusing thing about these symptoms that is definitely worth mentioning is that they may often be associated with other gastrointestinal disorders.* These symptoms usually come about in conjunction with some of the other symptoms listed above, so it's important to keep an eye on the big picture and to look for patterns.

EVERYBODY IS DIFFERENT

It's important to remember that as with any other health condition or disease, acid reflux is different for everybody. Though the symptoms listed above cover some of the more common that appears in individuals with acid reflux, there may be others that appear at any point in time. A person's age, lifestyle, family history, or other medical conditions may contribute to how acid reflux appears and takes hold.

In an infant for example, acid reflux may commonly be associated with fits of crying and even projectile vomiting. *It's important for parents to keep tuned to any difficulties with eating or unusual patters of vomiting that seem to be different than the usual baby spit up. In individuals that already have asthma, acid reflux may appear and tend to aggravate this condition.* This may result in such individuals having trouble breathing or going into asthma attacks in extreme cases as the stomach acid may only further complicate this already difficult condition.

The bottom line is that everybody is different, which is to say that sometimes the symptoms may show up in a more extreme state and sometimes it may not be quite as intense. *Some people may only suffer from one of the symptoms, while others may have an entire combination of symptoms. As an individual it's important to keep an eye on the symptoms that you do suffer from.* It can even be helpful to keep a journal noting when the symptoms occur, what they are, and when they tend to worsen.

Look for patterns of frequency or intensity to determine what is going on, as this may be a first step that you take with a doctor. Above all, get into a doctor to get proper diagnosis. This may be something that your general practitioner can help with, or it may be something that you require additional help with from a specialist if it is a more extreme case.

Start with your regular doctor and tell them about your symptoms, speak to when they get worse or how often you see them show up. If you take the initiative to go in with a bit of baseline education, then that can help your doctor with a proper diagnosis and ultimately treatment—because after all that's what you want so that you can live with and properly cope with this disease.

Every case of acid reflux is different so it's important to remember that and take matters into your own hands to help with an effective diagnosis and treatment plan.

COMMON SITUATIONS CAN AGGRAVATE THE CONDITION

What you may not realize is that certain conditions, factors, or items may tend to aggravate the acid reflux. *There are times when acid reflux may come on without question, and then there are circumstances where it may worsen as an already existing condition. Here are a few instances where you can expect to really suffer from or have a worse reaction to already existing acid reflux:*

Pregnancy: It is quite common that pregnant women may develop acid reflux. As the baby grows and the uterus grows along with it, this may tend to push on other organs.

This may ultimately result in an improper digestion of food or stomach acid backing up into the esophagus. Heartburn is a common symptoms of pregnancy and acid reflux is a condition that often develops as a result of pregnancy. It may go away after delivery or may continue on well after the baby is born.

Eating Big Meals: Let's face it; all of us have had a bit of indigestion after eating Thanksgiving dinner or other big meals. However for those who suffer from acid reflux, eating a big meal may send their symptoms into orbit. *The overconsumption of food may result in their inability to digest this, and the backup of stomach acids may be intensified. This is something to keep an eye on, and we'll discuss in later chapters how smaller meals more frequently can really help those with acid reflux.*

Trigger Foods: We will get into the specifics on foods and diet as they relate to acid reflux, as there's a lot to cover. It is worth noting though that certain foods may tend to further aggravate the condition and cause the symptoms to really come about fast and furiously. Sometimes you may not even realize that you have "trigger foods" until you start to really keep an eye on things closely. Understanding what works against you or makes things worse can really help to shed some light on how to cope with acid reflux.

Lifestyle and Habits: Certain habits such as smoking may tend to make the symptoms of acid reflux far worse. We know that these habits aren't good for us, but they can tend to make the condition much worse and the symptoms become far more prevalent.

You may find that you need to switch up your lifestyle as well because the simple act of lying down right after eating can cause you to really suffer. We will get into this further when we discuss how to live with acid reflux, but suffice it to say that you may need to make some changes in the long run.

Other Health Conditions: Suffice it to say that if you suffer from other health conditions, acid reflux may become far more likely. Adding to that the fact that certain gastrointestinal disorders such as a hiatal hernia where the stomach protrudes a bit up into the chest through the diaphragm may result in acid reflux.

Other conditions such as ulcers tend to go hand in hand with this condition. So if you suffer from other health conditions, keep an eye out for the common symptoms as acid reflux may become inevitable.

BEING EDUCATED CAN REALLY HELP

Though everybody is different when it comes to this often frustrating disorder, it's important to be educated. Understanding what can contribute to acid reflux showing up and more importantly how it can affect your life through common symptoms can help you to become educated and grab a hold of this disease.

You really are in the driver's seat and if you know what to look for and are in tune to any commonalities or symptoms to look for, then you will know how to better cope with the disease. Doctors welcome an educated patient, but remember that they are your best source for proper diagnosis and more importantly a treatment plan that works best for your individual needs.

Now you've seen what causes or contributes to acid reflux. You've seen what it looks like and know what acid reflux can do to you. Take this education and apply it to your life, and become educated to help get the help you really need. Next it's important to understand what to eat and how to live with acid reflux—and we will help you through that as well.

CHAPTER 3- A PROPER DIET FOR ACID REFLUX

Though maintaining a proper diet is important in just about every health condition, it's crucial as it relates to acid reflux. The foods that you eat may make things worse. There are even trigger foods that may be the very source of this awful health condition for you. You may not realize just how important your diet is to getting the necessary help required for acid reflux.

This is often overlooked as a cause for acid reflux, but the foods that you eat or don't eat can make a huge difference in how you cope with acid reflux and how bad it really gets. For some people, they may only have one or two trigger foods. For others, they may need to make an entire dietary change to focus in on foods that prevent them from having flare-ups that are commonly associated with acid reflux.

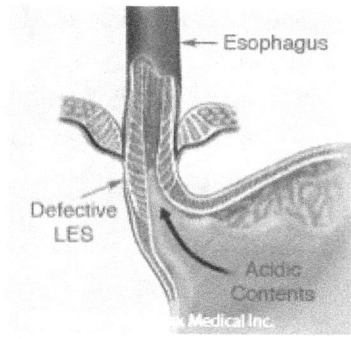

A defective LES, allows reflux back into the esophagus

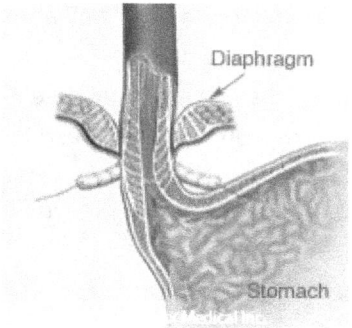

The LINX™ device is placed around the LES during a laparoscopic procedure

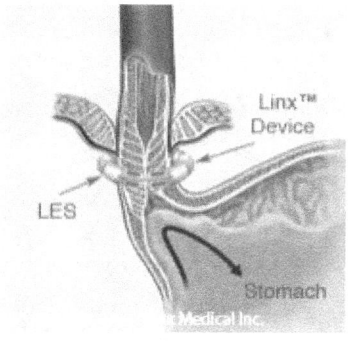

The LINX™ device is designed to "augment" the LES to prevent reflux

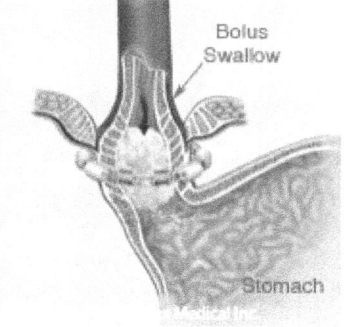

The LINX™ device is designed to accommodate normal swallow function

While it only makes sense that certain foods may tend to aggravate acid reflux and cause the symptoms to flare up, it can be more extreme for some. *It may feel as though every food causes some symptom to come about and this can be much to the detriment of those who have to live with acid reflux.* So where do you start? How do you know what foods are off limits and which ones are okay? It's important to remember that again acid reflux is different for everybody. The foods that cause major problems in some people may not even cause a reaction at all in other people. There are no two cases that are idertical. For some people it's all about the foods that they eat and for others it's all about about the portions. Some people may be able to eat whatever they want, but have to watch what they drink. While others suffer from more lifestyle factors that can trigger the symptoms—it just goes to show that acid reflux is truly different for everybody that experiences and suffer from it.

COMMON TRIGGER FOODS

Though there can an even longer list than we will portray, these cover the more common trigger foods. This list represents the foods that many people tend to complain of or have issues with. *These are foods that for some reason or another may tend to aggravate, hurt, or cause acid reflux to show up over and over again. So let's get into the list of common trigger foods as a starting point. Common trigger foods include:*

Spicy Foods: This can cover everything from a high dose of black pepper all the way up to cayenne or chili peppers. It may cover entire types of cuisine such as Mexican or Indian or it may be limited to a specific spice. For many who suffer from acid reflux, spicy foods in one form or another may tend to aggravate the condition and lead to the onset of symptoms that plague them.

Garlc: *Though garlic is certainly at the heart of many different home remedies, it may also tend to bring on symptoms of acid reflux for some. This could start off as simple heartburn and then run the gamut of symptoms from there.* This can range from foods that are made with garlic or be more specific such as eating garlic by itself.

Citrus Fruits: Due to their high acid content, citrus fruits are quite common as an irritant. Eating fruits such as oranges, pineapple, grapefruits, or even a squeeze of lemon or lime can cause some people to feel the burn almost immediately.

Fried Foods: This is a common one and it has as much to do with the fat content as the breading and preparation method. Any type of fried food may cause a person to immediately feel heartburn and this can quickly turn into more extreme symptoms. This is often a first food that doctors look to in understanding if trigger foods are responsible for an individual's symptoms of acid reflux.

Vinegar: You know that tart sensation that vinegar gives you, sometimes even from the smell? Well that acidity or tartness is a common culprit for those that suffer from acid reflux. This may be limited to using vinegar as a condiment or may appear as a more extreme case where an individual must avoid anything made with vinegar.

Tomatoes: Along the same lines as citrus fruits, tomatoes tend to have a high acidity content. This may be limited to tomatoes in their raw form, or may include tomato products such as ketchup, tomato sauce, tomato juice, or other products that use tomatoes as their basis.

Cruciferous Vegetables: *The very vegetables that are often the best for us can tend to cause gas. This may be common in those who don't even suffer from acid reflux as it's specific to these cruciferous vegetables.* For those that suffer from acid reflux, eating any of these vegetables such as cauliflower, broccoli, cabbage, or Brussels sprouts can cause some serious side effects.

Beans: Another trigger food that many people can point to is beans, and oftentimes it may be in any form. As there are many different types and variations of beans, this may be an area that people really need to focus on.

Caffeine: Though it works well to wake you up in the morning or give you that afternoon jump, caffeine can be off limits for those with acid reflux. This stimulant can cause the symptoms for some patients with acid reflux to flare up almost instantly. This is most commonly found with coffee directly, but may come up with tea, hot cocoa, or even chocolate.

Alcohol: *Though many people may try to ignore this trigger food, alcohol can cause some serious damage to those who suffer from acid reflux. The backup of stomach acid may be felt rather quickly or may not show up until the next day, but this is one trigger food to keep your eye on.*

So how do you know if you have problems with one trigger food over another? Unfortunately you may only be able to tell through trial and error and over time. This is where keeping a food journal may help. You may even develop problems with some of these trigger foods later on after your acid reflux has already been diagnosed.

Just as the symptoms of acid reflux may change over time, so too may the triggers that set it off. Your symptoms may have more to do with lifestyle factors, and we will get into coping with those in a later chapter. For now though, this comprehensive list supplies you with some of the more common trigger foods that you may expect to cause some sort of symptom of acid reflux.

WHAT DOES A PROPER DIET REALLY LOOK LIKE?

So we've seen what foods are common in terms of aggravating your symptoms. We've gone through what common trigger foods are, and what problems they can create. It can all be quite confusing as many people aren't sure exactly what they should eat. Part of this is focusing on the proper ways to eat, and we'll cover that in a later chapter where we look at necessary lifestyle changes.

You may feel as though you don't know where to start, or you may even be afraid of eating foods for fear of a reaction. Don't live in that fear! Know that some foods may present problems and others may not, even within one food group.

Know that some foods may be just fine at one time, and then may send you into orbit later on. *Acid reflux can be a very challenging health condition for many people as it may change shape or form along the way. So understanding what a proper diet may look like can at least help to provide a guideline*. This guideline will at least show you what healthy eating should look like in the first place—and we should all be striving for that as a practice anyhow.

Starting with the basics, here are some guidelines for a proper diet for those patients with acid reflux:

Fresh Fruits and Vegetables: If you've never had any problems with any sort of fruits or vegetables before, then the sky is the limit. Fresh fruits and vegetables provide necessary vitamins and nutrients that our bodies crave. They are low in calories and provide fiber in the process. All of these things are good and of course essential. If you're worried, then go slow with the cruciferous variety such as broccoli, cauliflower, and cabbage.

Always go for the cooked variety as raw tend to be harder to digest and tend to create more problems even for those who don't suffer from acid reflux. Start slow with the citrus fruits or vegetables in question and add to the list if they don't seem to present any problems. If you do find that these are the source of your triggers, then work to find substitutions that you can tolerate so that you can still get in your quota of nutrients throughout a day.

Whole Grains: *Though making the initial switch to whole grains may be hard, it can not only be good for your health but also good for your acid reflux as well. Sometimes starchy varieties of pasta, bread and rice can tend to aggravate acid reflux symptoms—not only that but they offer little or no nutritional value.*

Rather than eating white bread, pasta, or rice which offer high amounts of starch but little nutrition, turn to their whole grain counterparts. These are loaded with fiber and essential nutrients which may even help to ward off your symptoms. As with anything with fiber, make the transition slowly to avoid potential problems along the way.

Lean Protein: Many that suffer with acid reflux may find that fatty meats can tend to cause major heartburn and trigger other symptoms. As part of a healthy diet, you should avoid fatty meats anyhow but it's a good idea for acid reflux sufferers.

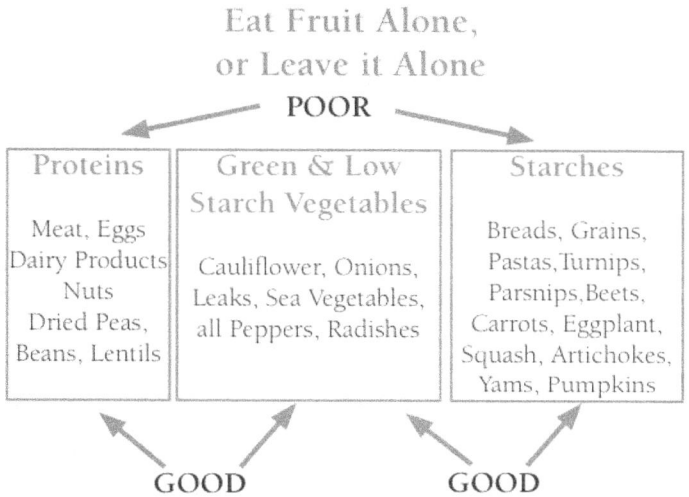

Eat Fruit Alone,
or Leave it Alone

POOR

Proteins	Green & Low Starch Vegetables	Starches
Meat, Eggs Dairy Products Nuts Dried Peas, Beans, Lentils	Cauliflower, Onions, Leaks, Sea Vegetables, all Peppers, Radishes	Breads, Grains, Pastas, Turnips, Parsnips, Beets, Carrots, Eggplant, Squash, Artichokes, Yams, Pumpkins

GOOD   GOOD

Get rid of the high fat or processed meats such as hot dogs, salami, bologna, or other types of processed lunch meats. Go for options such as lean ground beef, turkey, chicken, fish, and trim all visible fat off of meat that you eat. Try out tofu as a nice protein substitution and limit your meat intake, replacing red meat with poultry when you can.

Dairy Products: Though dairy can tend to cause problems for those that are lactose intolerant, they don't often show up on the list of possible suspects for those with acid reflux. Milk can help to neutralize stomach acids and can therefore be a big help. If you want to be sure though, start off slow and go with low fat options. Low fat milk, cottage cheese, yogurt, cheese, and sour cream are not only safer bets as they relate to acid reflux but may be of great help to a healthy lifestyle as well.

Beverages: *This may not seem like that important of a category, but it can really make a difference in how you live with acid reflux. Everything from caffeinated beverages to fizzy drinks can tend to cause problems, so approach this category with caution.* Of course water is the very best option, but if you're going to go with juice try the clear variety like apple or white grape—orange juice or even red grape juice can cause problems with acid reflux sufferers. Replace coffee with herbal or green tea as a substitute if necessary. Get rid of soda pop and instead try mineral water. If you must drink alcoholic beverages, try a white wine or clear alcohol such as vodka.

Fats: *We all enjoy snacks or fats of some kind at some point in time or another. Try lower fat versions of fatty treats, like low fat cookies or cakes made with applesauce instead of oils or butter. Try unsalted nuts rather than popcorn or replace junk food with healthier options.* The high fat content can really take a beating on your acid reflux, so choose your snacks wisely. When it comes to cooking, go for healthier oils such as olive oil as they offer health benefits and don't often result in problems for those with acid reflux.

LEARNING TO MODIFY ALONG THE WAY

There will be certain foods that are just fine for you and others that are off limits from the start. It's your job as the individual suffering from acid reflux to understand and establish which foods are okay for your system and which tend to present major problems.

This will come with time, and unfortunately involve a bit of potentially painful trial and error. Don't be afraid of an entire food group unless you know for certain that it presents problems. Before you assume that certain foods are certainly going to cause pain and discomfort, try them out. Know too that some foods will change and may affect you one day but not the next—that's the nature of acid reflux.

Learning to target the foods that are helpful and not harmful is part of learning to live with the disease. You will figure it out through time and will find the most effective way to cope and live with it. Part of the whole process is determining what if any lifestyle changes are required, and that's where we'll head to next on our journey for education for acid reflux.

CHAPTER 4- IMPORTANT LIFESTYLE CHANGES FOR ACID REFLUX

So you know what causes it, and you understand what the common symptoms are. You see how all of this can affect your life and are learning to focus in on the triggers that may cause problems for you. You have an excellent foundation and even understand what a proper diet should look like for acid reflux.

Now what, what could possibly be next in the process? When it comes to living with acid reflux, you will find that there are some rather important lifestyle changes. These can help to shape the way in which you cope with acid reflux and allow you to live a more enjoyable life. Though these may initially be thought of as sacrifices, over time you will see that the temporary frustration or discomfort that these modifications may cause can result in long term gain.

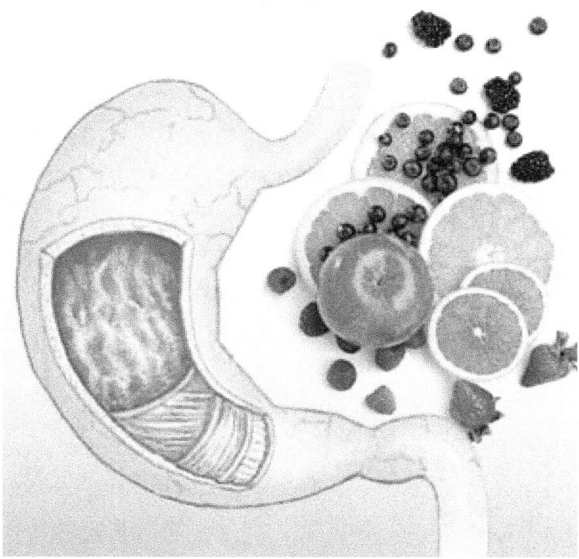

Learning how to live with acid reflux means taking a long hard look at the life you lead and looking for areas of potential change to make things more tolerable. You may be surprised at what some of these lifestyle changes involve.

You may find that most of them are things that you've thought of doing, but simply aren't. You may find that some of these things sound so impossible to get rid of or adapt that you may be inclined to look for another route. *These are the harsh realities and though you may not want to hear it, these lifestyle changes can make the difference between you being in a constant state of pain and suffering or you living successfully with the disease.*

COMMON LIFESTYLE CHANGES WORTH CONSIDERING

So what are these lifestyle changes? What do they involve and do you have to make all of these changes? Take a look for yourself at some of the more common lifestyle changes that can make a true impact in living with acid reflux. These include:

Eating Smaller Meals: Rather than diving into three huge meals a day, it can be quite helpful to break them into smaller meals more frequently throughout the course of a day. *This causes less strain on the digestive tract and this means far less likely of a possibility of stomach acid backing up into the esophagus. Break up your meals into smaller and more digestible ones, and this will even help with a healthier way of living in the process.*

Avoid Laying Down After Eating: The rule of thumb is that you shouldn't lie down within two hours of eating a meal. This allows you to be upright and aids in digestion, and this all contributes to the stomach acids staying where they are supposed to.

If you lay down after eating a meal, you are allowing the potentially already weakened esophageal sphincter to open up and this results in the awful flow of stomach acids back up into the esophagus. Eat your meals at least two hours before bedtime and do your part to avoid taking a nap within two hours of eating throughout the course of a day.

Quit *Smoking: If you smoke, then quit! It's really as easy as that because it's the only surefire way of avoiding smoke from irritating your acid reflux. Even secondhand smoke can aggravate the condition, but by quitting smoking you are at least doing your part to discontinue the smoke from making matters worse.* Smoking can and often will cause the symptoms of acid reflux to flare up, so by quitting smoking you are doing your part to stop the cycle from continuing on.

Limit Your Alcohol: Many of us may enjoy indulging in an alcoholic beverage here and there; however this can tend to cause some irritation as it relates to acid reflux. It's a good idea to really limit your alcoholic intake or even eliminate it if you find that it's a trigger for your symptoms. If you must enjoy a beverage, then keep it to a minimum and find a clear alcohol that you can enjoy which is far less likely to cause problems.

Avoid Stress or Learn How to Cope With It: One of the most common triggers of acid reflux is stress. This can cause more problems than certain foods, and is often found to be the root cause or trigger of the condition. Stress can cause so many different health problems and in this instance, it can really tend to aggravate existing symptoms or lead to more intense or frequent flare ups.

Learning to avoid stress whenever possible or at the very least learn to cope with it can be quite valuable as it relates to acid reflux—and it's also good for the rest of your health and well being at the same time. Coping with the daily stress that comes your way is an important part of living with acid reflux.

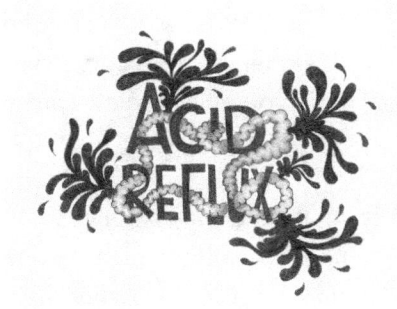

If it doesn't already act as a trigger, it very well might at some point in time, particularly if mixed with other potential culprits. This is one of the most important lifestyle adjustments to make in living successfully with acid reflux, so it's well worth looking at.

Keep Your Head Upright While You Sleep: Even if you work the rule of avoiding eating at least two hours before bedtime, acid reflux can work in mysterious ways. You may see a flare up come about just by the way you sleep and if you're not elevated enough, then this can lead to some major problems down the road. Do your part by sleeping slightly elevated, even if it's just by using an extra pillow to help things flowing as they should—this can make a huge difference in your sleep and your entire day.

Maintain a Healthy Weight: In all honesty, obesity can not only contribute to the likelihood of acid reflux but can make it worse. *When you are overweight, especially at extreme measures, then this puts a strain on your whole system. This may even contribute to the weakening of the esophageal sphincter in the first place, and can certainly weaken it more over time.*

If you are overweight this may even cause your other organs to push up on your stomach or put things out of line and this can cause additional aggravation and contribute to the symptoms of acid reflux. Keep your weight at a healthy range because this will avoid the problem. If you already suffer from acid reflux, then do your part to get your weight back to a healthy range and you will avoid further problems or symptoms.

This may be a difficult lifestyle change to make and may involve some major changes and sacrifices, but maintaining a healthy weight is one of the best ways to keep your acid reflux under control—or even help to get rid of it altogether in some instances.

Keep a Close Eye on Your Diet and Exercise: You now know what a healthy diet looks like when it comes to living with acid reflux. It's up to you to manage your diet and keep an eye on potential trigger foods.

You have to stay in control of your eating habits and always be tuned into the foods that may bother you. It's up to you to recognize when you've eaten too much and how to keep your portions and eating habits under control. As part of a healthy lifestyle, you should also have a strong focus on exercise.

Though exercise directly may not help to clear up or get rid of acid reflux, it can certainly help you to keep your weight at a healthy level and of course maintain better health overall. This is all part of the big picture and these are the necessary lifestyle changes that must be made to live comfortably and successfully with acid reflux.

One of the most important elements in dealing with and successfully living with acid reflux is to make the necessary lifestyle change. We've listed out some of the major categories and most common changes, but only you know what you need to change moving forward. For some, it is the way in which they deal with and process stress.

For others, it may be the eating habits that they've maintained their entire lives. Living with acid reflux is all about learning and growing. The reality is that it's a "work in progress" because you will likely have to make more changes and adjustments along the way, and these will all help you to successfully cope with this sometimes frustrating disease.

It can't be stressed enough that this is a different disease for everybody and therefore the lifestyle coming into it equals a variety of different changes. Though many people may be resistant to make these changes at first, it is quickly realized that this action may be the only way to live pain free.

WILL YOU MAKE THE NECESSARY CHANGES?

When the symptoms are lighter or less prevalent, it is really easy for people to push it aside and ignore the necessity to change. *It's not to say that your lifestyle necessarily put you in the predicament of having acid reflux, but there are obviously many factors that may contribute to the likelihood of it developing.*

That being said, once the symptoms start to worsen or come on more frequently, people start to realize that change is necessary. Though there are few people that may suffer from acid reflux and may be doing all the right things with no possible change required, this is an exception to the rule.

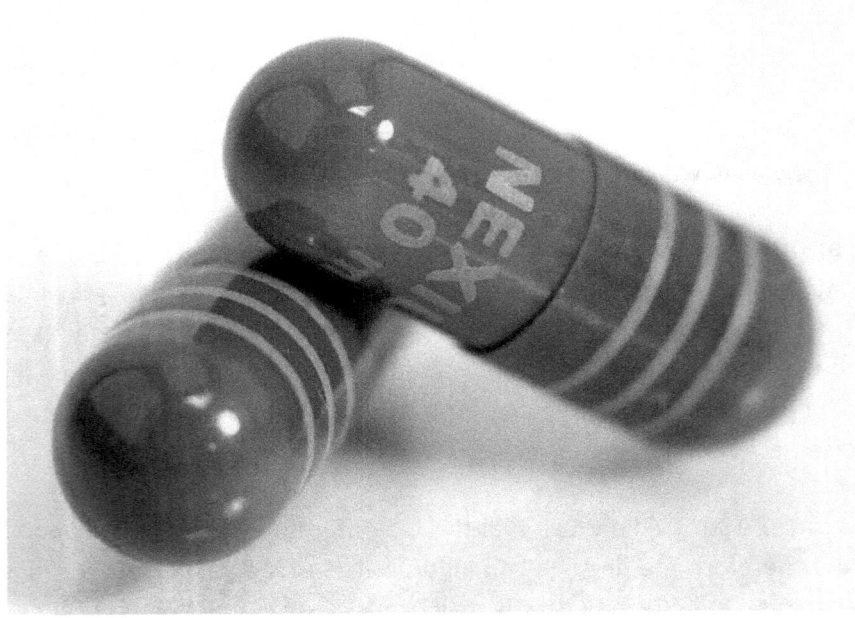

The majority of people who suffer from acid reflux can and should make some sort of change in their life. There is usually at least one area that can be changed which will lessen the symptoms and allow you to live more comfortably with acid reflux. The question is: will you make the necessary lifestyle changes?

Anytime you are asked to make lifestyle changes, it can be difficult. It can certainly mean sacrifice or difficulty in giving up the things that you are used to doing. Anytime you are asked to make a change it is met with resistance because you may like or be used to the way you do things. The problem is this—if you don't do something or make the changes required in your life, then the problem can worsen.

If you don't quit smoking or make the necessary changes in your diet, then you can expect the symptoms of acid reflux to get worse over time. *If you leave it alone and do nothing, the majority of the time acid reflux will worsen and become very frustrating and painful. If you want to avoid that pain and discomfort and somehow avoid a debilitating life because of acid reflux, then you will make the change.*

Take it slow at first and look at one major area at a time. See how much better you feel and adjust accordingly because again this is a "work in progress". Don't try to do it all at once, but just remember that the more willing you are to make the necessary changes and the more open you can have your eyes to your lifestyle, the better your chances are for living with acid reflux. You are in the driver's seat and if you work to overcome the obstacles that may worsen or contribute to your acid reflux, then you will find a way to live with it in a much better way.

Chapter 5- Options For Treating And Living With Acid Reflux

No matter what sort of lifestyle changes you may make or foods you may eat or avoid, the symptoms may still be there. The frustrating part of acid reflux is that it can change without any warning and the foods that were just fine one day become off limits the next.

This is a constantly changing disease and therefore you need to keep up with it. As we've discussed, the bulk of the responsibility is on you to keep tuned into the foods that you eat and the lifestyle that you lead to manage this disease.

That part will never change because you are always at the core of how you live with this disease. Additionally it's up to you to keep a food journal and take all of the necessary steps to stay well. Sometimes however it's just not enough! Sometimes you need some sort of treatment, whether it be medication or something more natural. Sometimes you need additional help above and beyond what you are capable of handling.

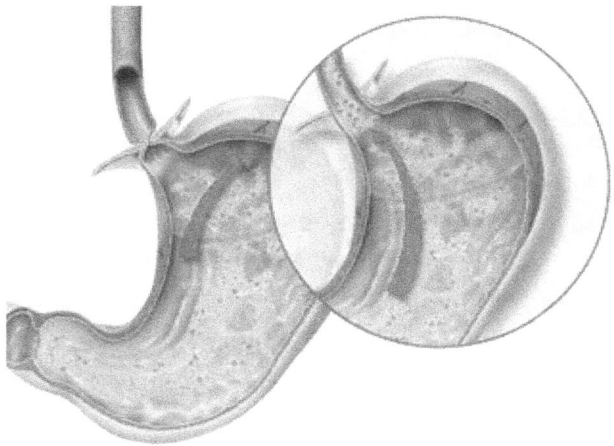

Your doctor is the best and most important person to decide upon your necessary treatment plan. However you play an active role in it because you need to decide when things aren't working or if changes are required. Only you know what's going on throughout the course of a day or week, and therefore your doctor may very well rely on you to inform them of what is going on with you.

If your symptoms worsen, become more frequent, or medication or prescribed treatment just isn't working, then you need to be the one to recognize that and work with your doctor to take the necessary next steps. For some people, they may get on a medication and stay on it for years without ever having to worry about it again.

These people have specific symptoms and may find that certain medications work well for them over the course of time. For others however, they may start out with natural or home remedies and then make the switch to prescription medication—the opposite situation may even occur. So you see yet again just how different acid reflux is in different people and how it truly is an individual disease. You see quickly that there is no "one size fits all" treatment plan.

WHAT ARE THE COMMON MEDICATIONS USED TO TREAT ACID REFLUX?

For as many different symptoms of acid reflux as there are out there, you can find just about as many medications. You can simply check your local pharmacy to see just how many products line the shelves with the promise of helping to solve your indigestion or reflux. So how do you make sense out it all? We won't get into the science of it all, but here are a few major categories of medications that can be of great help.

Antacids: *This is the most common medication that people turn to, particularly at the beginning. When people suffer from isolated incidents of heartburn or indigestion, they likely turn to some form of antacids.* These may help for awhile but if your symptoms worsen or as the acid reflux becomes more serious and more pronounced, these won't often offer the same level of relief. It's not to say that these will hurt you, but they will not necessarily offer you the same relief that they once did because they aren't as effective as your symptoms require.

Over-the-Counter Medications: This covers a very wide range of medications. Some come in the form of liquids, others come in the form of tablets, some you take before a meal, and others you take just after a meal—so you can get lost in the rows of various medications.

If your symptoms are new or if you have a mild case and simply want to try out an over-the-counter type of medication, then zero in on what your symptoms are and look for the medications that seem to offer the best relief. *Some medications that were once only offered through a prescription can now be found as over-the-counter varieties.* For example, you can find a milder version of Prilosec which has offered relief to acid reflux sufferers for years. This may be a good place to start and see how the over-the-counter medications work at relieving your symptoms.

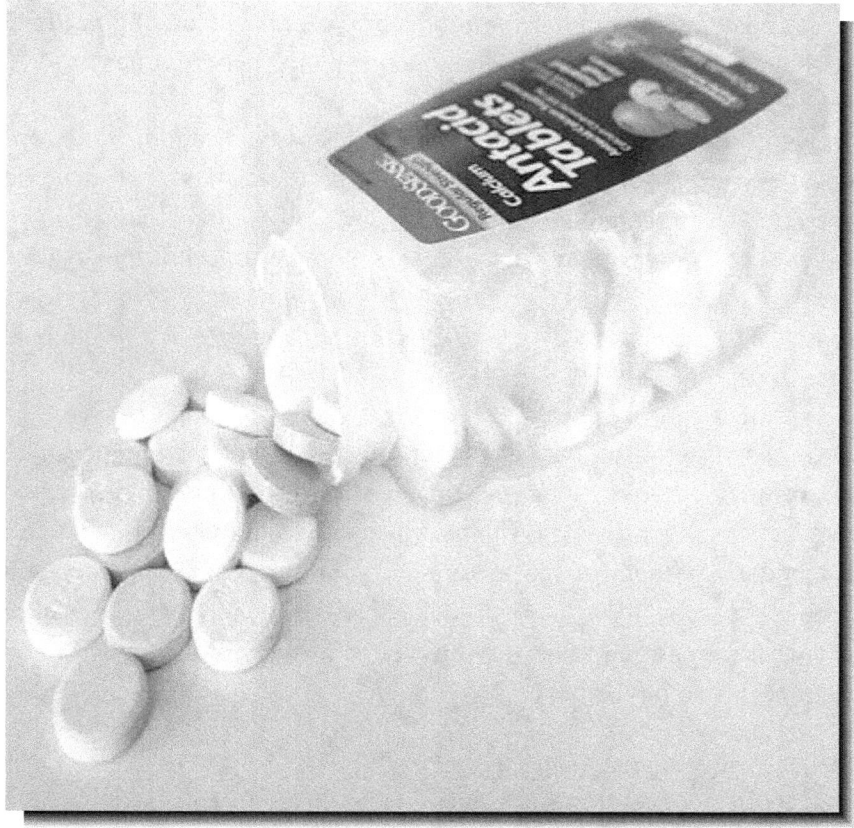

Prescription Medications: *These are bound to be a bit more potent, and are prescribed by doctors to deal with your specific symptoms. You may be put on an acid or "H2" blocker that actually slows or stops the production of stomach acid.* You may be put on anti-spasm medication that work to reduce the actual muscle spasms that may contribute to or even cause the acid reflux or backup of acid in the first place. You may be put on proton-pump inhibitor (PPI) which goes to work on the actual molecules responsible for the production of stomach acids. The type of prescription medication that you are put on has a lot to do with the severity, type, and frequency of your symptoms. Anything you have done to keep track of your symptoms or patterns will be of great help so that your doctor can work with you on an effective treatment.

Though these are only the major categories of medications, there are obviously many different combinations and varieties that may be prescribed or recommended. *Start slow if you are only beginning to experience light symptoms. Over-the-counter medications can work well if you are only beginning to experience symptoms, if the symptoms are minor or widespread, or if your doctor tells you that you have a mild case of acid reflux.*

If nothing seems to be helping or if your symptoms seem to be intensifying, then it may be time to turn to some prescription medications. Your doctor is the best judge of what may work best, but it's important that you be in tune to your symptoms and that you properly convey them at your visit. This is the only way to ensure proper treatment and find the most effective way of coping with and living with acid reflux.

WHAT ABOUT NATURAL REMEDIES?

In recent years, it has become quite popular to look at alternative ways of healing. This isn't specific just to acid reflux, but to all sorts of health conditions. Though some diseases or health conditions warrant the need to take prescription medication on a daily basis for proper treatment, there are certain conditions where you may be able to try some more natural or alternative types of treatment. Some patients may benefit from this method of coping with their symptoms. It may not work for everyone, and this may not be a methodology that all patients believe in, but it's well worth mentioning. *If you are resistant to taking medication on a daily basis or want to try out a more natural treatment, talk to your doctor about it. Though it may not work with every case of acid reflux, for some it may offer a nice alternative.* Your doctor can best gauge if these methods will work for you, but being educated is part of your responsibility in dealing with acid reflux. Here are a few of the natural or alternative types of treatments that may work well for some acid reflux sufferers:

Acupuncture: Though this is a relatively new practice within our culture, it has been around for centuries. Acupuncture uses tiny needles on your pressure points to help you cope with any ailments or pain that you may be having.

A licensed acupuncturist works with you by placing needles at the source of the pain or potential blockage that may be contributing to your health condition or ailment. *This requires an open mind on the part of the patient because it is different than any other type of traditional medicine, but some acid reflux sufferers may find some sort of relief by trying this method of healing.* It may require a few treatments to see results, but it can work for some people.

Herbal Therapy: This should be done in conjunction with your doctor and/or a professional that can point you towards the right types of herbs and of course the appropriate dosage. There are some herbs such as ginger, chamomile, and meadowsweet that have natural healing properties.

This can be quite helpful in getting rid of the symptoms or at least lessening their occurrence. Though these herbs can be quite helpful to some people, it's really important to have assistance from a trained professional as to which ones will work best for you. You want to be sure you know what each herb can offer, what the proper dosage is, and what specifically it can help with. Some patients who suffer from acid reflux may find that herbal therapy either on its own or when combined with acupuncture can provide great relief from their symptoms. Yet again though, this may not work for everybody.

Home Remedies: *The merit of these home remedies may be questionable, but they are worth mentioning. There are certain foods that you may find in your own home that are believed to be of great help.* Though some doctors may not necessarily prescribe these, they may not hurt to try.

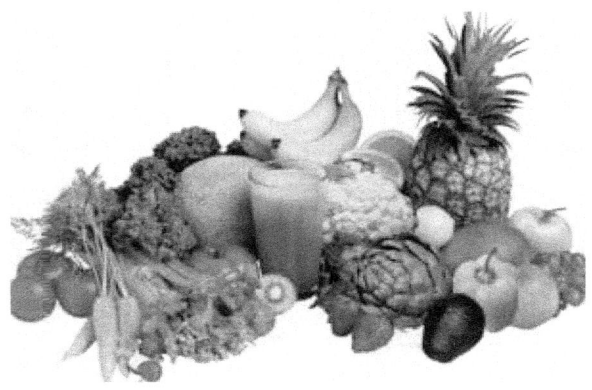

These can be especially helpful for those who have milder symptoms or for those who just want to turn to an alternative method to see what help it can bring. *Eating foods such as fresh papaya, fresh ginger, and marshmallow may provide great relief. They have natural healing properties that may help in coping with acid reflux and temporarily relieving the symptoms.* As with your regular diet, you may have to play around with the foods that help, but they can't hurt to try for a natural way of healing.

A TREATMENT FOR EVERYONE

As with every other aspect of acid reflux, it is a very individual disease. Those who suffer from it are the best gauge of the types of symptoms that they have, as well as the severity and frequency for which they occur. In some instances, natural treatments may be the best option and may offer great relief.

In other cases, where the symptoms are widespread or a bit milder, patients may find that over-the-counter medications are the very best option. *As acid reflux is such an individual disease, so too are the medications or treatment plans that offer the very best help. You as an individual are the best judge of what helps, and if you coordinate your doctor's guidelines and advice, you are sure to find the very best treatment for your symptoms.*

If at first you don't find relief from a particular treatment, then try another one. If you are sick of taking medication without any relief, then try a natural therapy. This is a disease for which treatment may grow and change with you as the symptoms vary. You may find a medication that you can stick with for the long haul and stay with for years which brings you the necessary relief.

Keep tuned into what is working and more importantly what is not. Do your due diligence to monitor and track what's going on and alter your treatment accordingly. It's important to do all of this under the supervision of a doctor, particularly because you don't want to move forward with improper medications or dosages.

Talk to your doctor and decide together what the very best treatment plan is for you, and if something isn't working look for the best alternatives. There are many different ways of treating acid reflux, and this makes it a health condition that you can live with. As you maintain control of your acid reflux, you are sure to find the very best treatment to help you find relief and some comfort in the process. There is truly something for everyone!

CHAPTER 6- CONCLUSION

We have provided you with all of the insight on acid reflux. We've taken you through the steps to understand how it occurs, what causes it, and what you can do to live with it. This is only part of the equation because education is the beginning and learning to live with it is the other important part. Being an educated patient and consumer can help you to find the appropriate treatments.

When it comes to acid reflux, education is an important aspect of living with it. If you take control of the disease, then it is sure to not take control of you. This is a health condition that you can effectively live with, and it is something for which treatment is not only available but is recommended. It's important for you to keep tuned into your symptoms and to see what is working and what is not.

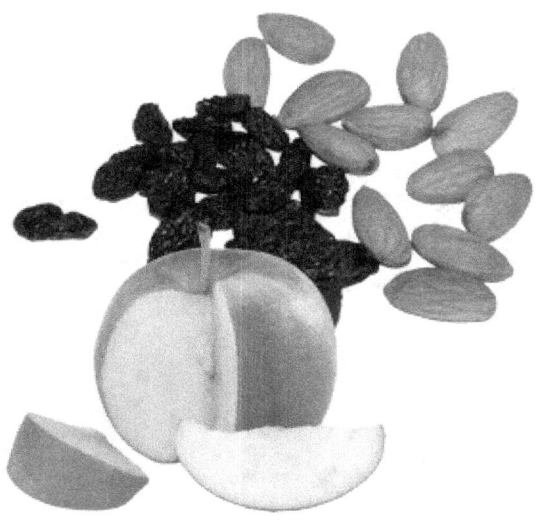

This is a health condition for which the foods you eat and the lifestyle that you lead can have a great effect on how you live with it. This is a very treatable health condition, but it takes your focus and insight to understand how acid reflux is affecting you. We've provided you with an understanding of what acid reflux is and how it works.

We've shown you how the symptoms may unveil themselves and how they may change over time. We've shown you what a proper diet looks like and even discussed what common trigger foods may be. We've indicated the different types of medications and treatments that there are out there.

Now the rest is up to you—because ultimately you are in the driver seta for how you live with this disease. You are the best indicator of how acid reflux is affecting you and more importantly how you can find the best way for living with it.

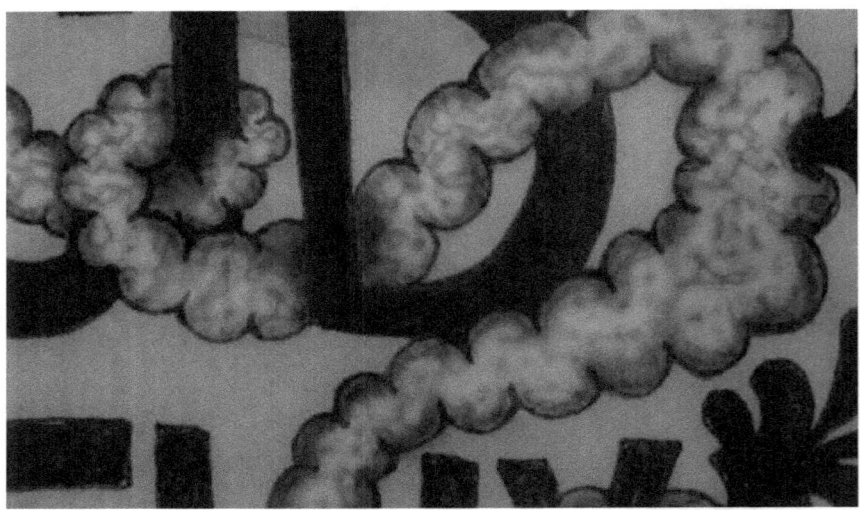

People live with acid reflux and find the most comfortable way to do so. Though it's been said before it bears repeating—this is a very individual disease. There is no "one size fits all" treatment just as there is no one way for which the disease shows itself. This can be a very livable health condition and if you stay in tune with all of the symptoms and how acid reflux presents itself within you, then you will live with it for years and likely not even give it a second thought.

Acid reflux doesn't have to rule your life, it only will if you let it. Though it is certainly a health condition to take seriously, it doesn't have to ruin you. You can lead a healthy lifestyle and you can make the necessary changes to make this health condition a bit more bearable.

Through time, you will find which treatment methods work best and what lifestyle fits your condition. You have all the tools to understand acid reflux, now it's up to you to do something about it. Living with acid reflux is very possible, and now you can take the necessary education to do something about it. Go forward, learn to live with acid reflux, and enjoy life again—the choice is up to you!

ABOUT THE AUTHOR

Brenda Suarez has inspired many individuals on how to be very creative. She has a lot of experience on the subject of Acid Reflux and has done extensive studies on this medical issue. Her continued involvement in the work associate with this medical problem has become very inspirational to persons who have an issue with their digestive system. This author has provided witty and engaging advice on ethics with respect to the Acid Reflux.

This author dispenses a lot of fabulous information about Acid Reflux. She has done exceptional work and studies on the problem which affects almost everyone in societies. Brenda continues to pursue and is committed to further studies in trying to help and offer great information with absolutely accuracy on the subject at hand

She is the author of several other books which gives detail information on specific topic in the medical world. She lives a happy and content life with her husband Nick Suarez and there three beautiful children.

www.ingramcontent.com/pod-product-compliance
Lightning Source LLC
Chambersburg PA
CBHW071355310526
45790CB00017B/1044